WALL PILATE FOR WOMEN OVER 50

Comprehensive Beginners fitness Exercise for Seniors to Lose Weight, Gain balance and Achieve good posture With Less Effort

Margaret A. Brinson

TABLE OF CONTENT

INTRODUCTION

A woman named Rose lived in Metropolis, a bustling metropolis where the pace of life frequently left little time for self-care. At the age of 50, she became involved in a web of everyday chores, ignoring her well-being in the middle of chaos.

The memories of her bright youth were overwhelmed by continuous pains in her neck and back, joints rebelling with every stride, and hips burdened by tension.

Rose's road to a transforming chapter began when she came across this book Wall Pilate for Women Over 50.

As Rose immersed herself in its pages, she found the healing power of Wall Pilates, a gentle but powerful workout regimen devised exclusively for women in their fifties.

The book's teachings unfolded like a road map, directing Rose through focused exercises that relieved her neck and back stiffness, reduced joint pain, and restored hip flexibility.

Rose, inspired by fresh information and a desire to break free from the chains of suffering, enthusiastically accepted the Wall Pilates routine.

With each attentive movement, she felt the weight of tension melt away, replaced by a sensation of power and renewal. The book became her valued friend, guiding her to a life free of health-related fears.

Rose is now a living example of Wall Pilates' effectiveness for ladies over the age of 50. Her life, which was formerly dominated by physical discomfort, has transformed into a beautiful tapestry of energy and fulfillment.

Through the prism of Rose's journey, the book offers a guiding light for women in their elder years, providing not just exercises but also a story of empowerment, resilience, hence creating the Life you desire.

Chapter 1: Understanding the benefits

Wall Pilates provides several benefits specialized exclusively for women over 50, addressing both physical and emotional well-being. This low-impact workout is a highly effective way to improve core strength, flexibility, and balance.

As women age, preserving these features becomes more important for their general health.

One significant advantage is better posture. Wall Pilates promotes appropriate spine alignment, which helps to mitigate the consequences of extended sitting and age-related bone density decreases.

Improved posture not only helps to give a more confident and youthful appearance, but it also relieves joint tension, lessening the discomfort commonly associated with aging.

Additionally, wall Pilates enhances joint mobility, focusing on regions that may get tight over time. This is especially advantageous for women over 50 who may suffer from arthritis or other joint problems.

The wall's regulated motions and modest resistance help to an expanded range of motion while reducing joint stress.

Another significant advantage is the emphasis on muscular tone. Wall Pilates works many muscle groups, assisting in the maintenance and growth of lean muscular mass.

This is critical for women in this age range because it helps counteract the natural reduction in muscle mass that comes with age. Maintaining muscular strength is critical for sustaining regular activity and avoiding injuries.

Beyond the physical advantages, Wall Pilates focuses on mindfulness and breathing techniques. This not only alleviates tension, but also improves mental clarity and concentration.

These components contribute to a comprehensive approach to well-being for women over the age of 50 who are dealing with menopause and hormonal changes.

Wall Pilates for women over 50 is a comprehensive training program that addresses core strength, flexibility, joint health, muscle toning, and mental wellness.

Incorporating this exercise into a daily routine can help women age gracefully, promoting a balanced and healthier lifestyle.

Tailoring exercises for women over 50

Tailoring workouts for women over 50 entails developing a fitness regimen that stresses flexibility, strength, and general wellness. Begin with dynamic warm-ups that include moderate stretches to get the body ready for more strenuous actions.

To improve cardiovascular health while avoiding joint pain, focus on low-impact exercises such as swimming or brisk walking.

Resistance exercise is essential for women over 50 in order to preserve muscle mass and bone density. Use resistance bands or modest weights to target main muscle groups.

Strengthening the core with planks and abdominal exercises improves stability and posture, which are important for this age range.

Balance exercises become more vital as we age. Include exercises like single-leg stands or Tai Chi to enhance balance and lessen the danger of falling.

Incorporating yoga or Tai chi helps relaxation and stress reduction, which improves general mental health.

To improve joint flexibility, prioritize stretching regimens that target regions prone to stiffness, such as the hips, shoulders, and spine. Yoga positions such as downward dog and cat-cow stretches might be useful.

Consider integrating exercises such as mild cycling or water aerobics to enhance joint mobility while minimizing impact.

Cardiovascular health is still a priority for women over the age of 50. Aerobic workouts like swimming or cycling are gentle on the joints. Interval training can also be beneficial, since it alternates between periods of greater intensity and rest.

Individual preferences and fitness levels differ. Customize the training regimen to your specific comfort and ability, gradually increasing intensity.

A consultation with a fitness expert or healthcare practitioner is recommended to ensure a safe and successful training program.

A well-rounded fitness program for women over 50 should include dynamic warm-ups, weight training, balancing exercises, joint-friendly aerobics, and flexibility routines.

Customizing the activity to meet individual demands guarantees a long-term and pleasurable approach to health and vitality.

importance of wall support

Wall support is critical for improving workout efficacy, particularly for women over 50 who do wall Pilates. The relevance of this support stems from its capacity to offer a firm foundation for correct alignment and balance throughout workouts.

As people age, maintaining stability becomes increasingly important for preventing accidents and supporting general well-being.

The wall acts as a stable anchor, allowing women over 50 to practice Pilates movements with confidence. It serves as a reference point, allowing for proper body alignment and lowering the danger of joint strain.

This is especially advantageous for people who have pre-existing ailments or worries about joint health, as wall support provides an extra degree of protection.

Wall support aids in the engagement of core muscles. Strengthening the core is critical for women over 50 in order to promote improved posture and prevent back issues that might occur as they age.

The wall provides consistent support, promoting perfect form and ensuring that the core muscles are utilized throughout the Pilates practice.

Furthermore, wall support enables a progressive rise in difficulty. Women over 50 may find certain Pilates movements difficult at first, but with the help of a wall, they may progressively improve their strength and flexibility.

This versatility is essential for customizing exercises to individual fitness levels, resulting in a safe and productive fitness journey.

Incorporating wall support into Pilates workouts promotes confidence and independence. Knowing there is a sturdy surface to rely on allows women over 50 to exert themselves without fear of losing balance.

This improved confidence not only improves the physical advantages of the workout, but it also helps to maintain a happy mood and general well-being.

Wall support is essential for ladies over 50 who do Pilates. It promotes stability, optimal muscular activation,

advancement, and a sense of confidence. Incorporating wall support into your training

program is a good investment in maintaining
health and energy as you age.

Chapter 2: foundations of wall pilates techniques

Wall Pilates techniques provide a unique and efficient approach to training, which is especially good for ladies over the age of 50. These fundamental exercises emphasize the use of a wall to improve stability, flexibility, and overall well-being.

This particular style of exercise, which incorporates Pilates principles, addresses the unique requirements and obstacles that elderly women confront.

Wall Pilates is built on a foundation of core strength. As women age, keeping a strong core becomes more important for stability and posture.

Wall Pilates works the abdominal muscles, lower back, and pelvic floor, helping to enhance balance and lessen the chance of injury. The wall serves as a prop, providing support and allowing people to move with appropriate form, resulting in a safe and successful workout.

Flexibility is another important aspect of Wall Pilates. Because joints grow less flexible with age, these approaches try to improve range of motion through controlled motions and stretches.

The wall acts as a guide, allowing for mild stretches that build flexibility in a supportive atmosphere. This is especially good for women over 50, who may develop stiffness or discomfort as they age.

Wall Pilates also emphasizes posture adjustment. The exercises focus on the muscles essential for maintaining an upright posture, counteracting the consequences of slouching or poor alignment.

This not only leads to a more confident image, but it also helps to prevent common problems like back discomfort and muscle imbalances.

Overall, Wall Pilates for women over 50 focuses on core strength, flexibility, and posture development.

The use of the wall as a support offers a safe and accessible workout, making it an excellent training option for people looking to maintain or improve their physical well-being as they age.

Exploring posture and alignment

Discovering proper posture and alignment is critical, especially for women over 50 who practice wall Pilates. As the body ages naturally, maintaining appropriate posture becomes increasingly important for general health.

Wall Pilates is a revolutionary training program that uses the vertical surface to improve alignment awareness. This technique enables ladies over 50 to achieve a harmonic balance of strength and flexibility.

Participants can improve their posture by methodically exercising muscles and increasing core stability and spinal alignment.

Exploration of posture within the Wall Pilates emphasizes conscious bodily awareness. Participants concentrate on aligning their spine, shoulders, and hips, which promotes a more upright posture. This not only promotes an elegant look, but it also lowers the danger of joint strain, which is usually connected with age.

Alignment, a critical part of this discipline, requires precise body placement. Women over the age of 50 can enhance their alignment by making intentional movements that promote muscle activation and joint mobility. This, in turn, promotes greater balance and lowers the risk of injury.

The Wall Pilates technique is unique in that it meets the special demands of women over 50. As people investigate their own alignment, they find the transforming potential of conscious movement.

This practice emphasizes the mind-body connection and promotes a holistic approach to physical well-being.

In essence, exploring posture and alignment with Wall Pilates allows women over 50 to take control of their bodies. It's more than simply a workout; it's a voyage of self-discovery that promotes resilience, strength, and a new feeling of life.

With each conscious movement, participants unleash the potential for better posture and alignment, pushing the boundaries of traditional exercise.

Breathing techniques for mature practitioners

As women mature, including mindful breathing methods into their workout regimens becomes increasingly crucial.

Focusing on breath control when doing wall Pilates for adult practitioners might improve the entire experience and benefits. Deep, focused breaths not only induce relaxation but also help to engage core muscles properly.

For women over 50, the Wall Pilates practice offers a one-of-a-kind opportunity to combine breath awareness with gentle yet powerful exercises.

Begin by breathing deeply through the nose, allowing the abdomen to expand, and then exhaling completely through pursed lips, clenching the core muscles. This regulated breathing complements Wall Pilates routines well, generating a mind-body connection that is both refreshing and empowering.

One of the primary benefits of mindful breathing in wall Pilates is the potential to improve spinal alignment.

As practitioners perform motions against the wall, synchronizing the breath with each action develops greater posture and spinal stability, both of which are critical for preserving general health and mobility as we age.

Furthermore, aware breathing helps to reduce stress, which improves mental health. Women over 50 endure several daily pressures, and including breath awareness into Wall Pilates creates a haven for mental calm.

This harmonic synthesis provides practitioners with not just physical strength, but also mental clarity and emotional stability.

In the domain of adult women's fitness, Wall Pilates stands out as a comprehensive discipline that addresses both physical and emotional well-being.

Practitioners who embrace conscious breathing methods in this setting open up a route to energy, strength, and tranquility.

As women traverse the complexities of age, Wall Pilates becomes a transforming trip in which breath serves as a silent guide, resulting in a harmonic integration of body and soul.

Customizing routines for individual needs

Tailoring training programs to individual requirements is critical, especially for women over 50 who participate in Wall Pilates.

Recognizing the specific needs of this group is critical for attaining the best results and encouraging overall well-being.

Women over 50 may have different fitness levels, health issues, and personal preferences.

 Customizing wall Pilates exercises enables tailored adaptations based on joint flexibility, muscle strength, and any existing physical restrictions.

This method assures that each session is not only beneficial but also safe and pleasurable.

Wall Pilates emphasizes core strength, and customisation allows for the introduction of exercises that especially target abdominal muscles, resulting in posture development and stability.

 For women in this age bracket, focusing on workouts that increase bone density becomes critical for general skeletal health.

Adjusting intensity levels is another important part of personalization. Progress should be gradual, taking into account aspects such as stamina and endurance.

Customized routines may include a combination of isometric and dynamic exercises, allowing people to push themselves without risking injury.

In addition to physical requirements, mental and emotional factors should not be disregarded. Routines may be tailored to meet personal tastes and goals, which increases motivation and adherence.

Incorporating mindfulness and relaxation methods into Wall Pilates workouts can help to reduce stress and enhance mental health.

Furthermore, understanding the value of variation is critical. Customized programs can add variety to workouts, avoiding boredom and activating different muscle areas.

This holistic approach is tailored to individual needs and provides a total exercise experience.

Customizing Wall Pilates routines for women over 50 is a deliberate strategy that considers physical fitness, emotional well-being, and individual preferences. By adapting workouts to individual needs, the advantages go beyond physical fitness and improve overall health and lifestyle.

Chapter 3: functional wall pilates movements

Functional wall Pilates exercises provide a refreshing approach to training, particularly for women over 50.

These exercises effortlessly combine Pilates principles with the assistance of a wall, resulting in a unique and effective training experience.

These routines, which focus on core strength, flexibility, and overall well-being, cater to the special demands of older women while fostering a balanced and healthy lifestyle.

The addition of a wall to Pilates exercises improves stability and allows for regulated movements, making it especially advantageous for people dealing with the problems of aging.

Engaging in these exercises against the wall provides a supporting surface, decreasing joint strain and increasing muscle engagement. This is especially important for women over 50 since it improves joint health and reduces the chance of injury.

Functional wall. Pilates techniques emphasize functional fitness by mirroring regular tasks. These exercises increase the body's capacity to accomplish daily chores with ease, which contributes to a higher quality of life.

As women age, retaining functioning and mobility becomes increasingly important, and these groups address this issue by encouraging elegant aging and greater vitality.
The adaptability of walls Pilates provides a full-body exercise by addressing many muscle groups at once. From easy stretches to specific core workouts, the wall is a

dependable companion in building total body strength. This comprehensive approach is particularly pertinent for women over 50 since it tackles the multiple facets of aging, encouraging a sense of empowerment and self-care.

Incorporating Functional Wall Incorporating Pilates into a training program for women over 50 promotes not just physical well-being but also mental and emotional health.

Pilates' focused nature promotes a mind-body connection, resulting in mental clarity and stress alleviation.

It evolves into a therapeutic practice that not only improves physical fitness but also fosters a happy outlook, making it an important component of the health path for women in their fifties and beyond.

Integrating functional exercises

When functional movements are incorporated into Wall Pilates programs, they have a significant impact on the well-being of women over 50.

These exercises emphasize motions that are similar to everyday tasks, therefore improving strength, flexibility, and balance.

Incorporating functional exercises into Wall Pilates sessions for this group provides a more comprehensive approach to fitness, addressing the specific demands of senior women.

Wall Pilates is known for its ability to enhance posture and core strength. Women over the age of 50 can improve their functional fitness by including functional activities into their routine. Squats against the wall, for example, focus not just the lower body but also the core muscles, resulting in increased stability.

Furthermore, including functional exercises into Wall Pilates sessions helps improve joint mobility, which is especially important for women in their fifties.

Leg swings and arm circles during wall-based Pilates workouts can assist maintain and develop flexibility, lowering the risk of injury and promoting general joint health.

The inclusion of functional exercises also provides cerebral stimulation, since participants participate in deliberate motions that correspond to real-world tasks.

This mental engagement is especially advantageous for women over 50, since it promotes both cognitive well-being and physical health.

Furthermore, functional workouts allow for individualization, catering to different fitness levels and goals.

Whether focused on balance, strength, or flexibility, the range of functional exercises in Wall Pilates sessions caters to the unique demands of women in this age group.

Integrating functional exercises with Wall Pilates for women over 50 results in a more holistic workout experience.

This combination not only addresses the fundamental concepts of Pilates, but also improves functional fitness, giving a well-rounded approach to health for older women who want to live an active and lively lifestyle.

Enhancing mobility and flexibility

As women age, maintaining mobility and flexibility becomes increasingly important for their general well-being.

Wall Pilates for women over 50 appears as a healthy and low-impact training option to address these difficulties.

This particular type of Pilates uses a wall for support, giving stability while increasing strength and flexibility.

One major advantage of Wall Pilates is its emphasis on core strength. As women age, their core muscles atrophy, resulting in lower back discomfort and diminished stability. Wall Pilates works the core with regulated movements, developing a strong and stable center. This not only helps to improve posture but also prevents injuries caused by weakening core muscles.

Wall Pilates also contains mild stretches and movements that especially target regions prone to stiffness, such as the hips and shoulders.

These motions help to enhance flexibility, which is essential for maintaining a complete range of motion throughout regular tasks.

Improved flexibility can reduce joint stiffness and increase general mobility, making daily chores easier for women over 50.

Furthermore, the usage of the wall in this Pilates variant adds another depth to the exercise.
It offers a support system that allows people to progressively ease into exercises, making it appropriate for those who are new to Pilates or have physical restrictions.

The wall serves as a guide, maintaining precise alignment and minimizing the possibility of strain.

Consistency is essential when implementing Wall Pilates into a training regimen. Regular practice can result in visible gains in mobility, flexibility, and general strength.

As women over 50 adopt this individualized Pilates method, they empower themselves to age gracefully while actively caring for their physical well-being.

Strengthening core muscles with wall support

Improving core strength is critical, especially for women over 50 looking for effective, low-impact activities. Wall support becomes an essential tool in this effort, providing stability and assisting with focused muscle engagement.

This method employs Pilates concepts, synchronizing breath and movement to strengthen the core while minimizing strain.

Wall-supported core workouts are designed to meet the specific needs of women in this age range, emphasizing safety and progressive growth.

Gentle yet forceful motions performed with the assistance of a wall reduce the chance of harm while increasing outcomes. Leg lifts, knee-to-chest stretches, and moderate twists against the wall are excellent workouts for activating abdominal muscles while minimizing joint stress.

These personalized exercises help to increase not just core strength but also posture and balance, which are important for general well-being.

As women age, these variables become more important in preventing injuries and encouraging a healthy, active lifestyle.

Furthermore, the wall functions as a variable prop, allowing for changes to match different fitness levels.

 Whether you're a novice or an experienced athlete, the wall can help you customize the intensity of your workout.

This flexibility promotes inclusion by making core strengthening available to a wide spectrum of women over 50.

Consistency is essential for receiving the advantages of wall-supported core workouts.

Integrating these activities into a regular training regimen not only promotes physical resilience, but also mental concentration and awareness.

Women who embrace the transformational potential of wall-supported core workouts enable themselves to age gracefully and vitally, embracing the essence of holistic well-being.

Chapter 4: Mind-body Connection in Wall Pilates

Wall Pilates provides a unique method to mind-body connection that is especially useful to ladies over the age of 50.

 This specialist version of Pilates focuses on using a wall to improve stability, flexibility, and strength.

The mind-body connection is essential to this practice because it teaches practitioners to be attentive to their movements, breathing, and total body awareness.

Maintaining a healthy mind-body connection becomes increasingly critical for women in their 50s and beyond in terms of general health.
Wall Pilates caters to this population by offering a supportive setting in which people may engage in exercises that not only increase physical strength but also promote mental clarity and awareness. The wall serves as a stabilizing factor, allowing

participants to concentrate on perfecting their moves without danger of imbalance or strain.

Mindful breathing is a key component of Wall Pilates, facilitating relaxation and stress reduction. As women age, stress management becomes increasingly important for their overall health.

Wall Pilates promotes deep, regulated breathing, resulting in a sensation of peace that benefits both the body and the mind.

Wall Pilates includes exercises that build core strength, which is essential for maintaining good posture, minimizing back discomfort, and supporting general spinal health.
This emphasis on the core goes beyond the physical sphere, as participants get a more acute awareness of their body's center, resulting in a harmonic link between the mind and muscles.

As women age into their 50s and beyond, joint flexibility becomes increasingly important. Wall Pilates tackles this by adding gentle stretches and motions to reduce stiffness and increase range of motion.

 The focused execution of these exercises strengthens the mind-body connection, resulting in a comprehensive approach to fitness customized to the unique demands of mature women.

To summarize, wall Pilates for women over 50 provides a dynamic combination of physical and emotional advantages.

The use of a supporting wall, along with a focus on mindful movements and breathing, promotes a deep mind-body connection that improves general well-being and energy.

Mindfulness practices During wall Pilates pilates

Incorporating mindfulness practices into Wall Pilates for Women Over 50 improves the whole experience by encouraging a harmonious connection between the mind and body.

As people age, it becomes increasingly important to prioritize their overall well-being, and mindfulness is a valuable tool for striking this balance.

The importance of breath awareness during Wall Pilates workouts cannot be overstated. Having participants coordinate their breath with each action generates a stronger sensation of presence.

Encourage deep, purposeful breathing to promote relaxation, reduce tension, and improve mental clarity. This attentive breathing method not only boosts the physical advantages of wall Pilates, but it also promotes a calm mental state.

Mindful movement is another essential component of the practice. Encouraging women over 50 to pay attention to the feelings in their bodies while performing various activities against the wall promotes a stronger mind-body connection.

This increased awareness enables participants to move with intention, resulting in improved posture, flexibility, and strength.

Wall Pilates provides unique chances for mindfulness via visual attention. The wall serves as a steady focus point, improving attention and helping to calm the mind.

Instructing participants to maintain visual concentration throughout exercises helps them be present in the moment, reducing distractions and fostering meditative states.

Furthermore, including small moments of rest and thought within the Wall Pilates exercise improves awareness.

Taking pauses to check in with the body, detect any tension, and make conscious modifications enables women over 50 to tailor the practice to their own requirements, promoting a more customized and thoughtful approach to Pilates.

Incorporating mindfulness techniques into Wall Pilates sessions for women over 50 improves the experience by boosting both physical and mental well-being.

This holistic approach encourages people to accept the mind-body link, which promotes overall health and vitality.

Mental health benefits for women over 50

As women age, prioritizing mental health becomes increasingly important, particularly for those over 50.

This era of life frequently presents unique obstacles, such as menopause, changes in family relationships, and significant health issues. Regular physical activity can considerably improve mental well-being.

Pilates exercises improve flexibility, strength, and balance, increasing overall physical health and offering a sense of success.

Social ties are crucial for mental health, and women over 50 can benefit from developing meaningful relationships. Participating in group activities, joining groups, or volunteering might help you build social links and reduce feelings of loneliness. This sense of community promotes a good attitude and emotional resiliency.

Mindfulness activities, such as meditation and deep breathing exercises, are effective tools for stress and anxiety management. Women of this age might find peace in mindfulness, which increases self-awareness and promotes emotional stability.

Staying present in the moment allows you to negotiate life's changes more easily.

Continued learning and following hobbies give mental stimulation, which helps to prevent cognitive degeneration.

Intellectual engagement, whether by learning a new language, playing a musical instrument, or diving into literature, keeps the mind sharp and develops a sense of fulfillment.

Developing a good sleep schedule is critical for mental wellness. Women over the age of 50 should emphasize enough and high-quality sleep, since it has a direct influence on mood, cognitive function, and general health.

Adequate rest improves emotional resilience and helps manage everyday pressures more efficiently.

Obtaining professional help via therapy or counseling might be beneficial. Open conversation about mental health issues is critical, and seeking professional help may provide helpful coping methods and emotional support.

Prioritizing mental health for women over 50 entails a comprehensive approach that includes physical exercise, social relationships, mindfulness, ongoing learning, enough sleep, and seeking professional help.

Incorporating these factors into daily life helps build a good and resilient mentality, improving overall well-being at this time of life.

Building Inner Strength Through Mindful Movements

Building inner strength through mindful exercises is a transformative experience, particularly for women over 50.

Engaging in disciplines such as wall Pilates not only improves physical health but also builds mental resilience.

Wall Pilates' blend of regulated movements and mindful breathing results in a harmonic synergy that fosters a profound connection between the mind and body.

Mindful movements, like those used in Wall Pilates, encourage practitioners to concentrate on the present moment.

This purposeful concentration cultivates a higher level of awareness, allowing people to access their inner strength.

As women negotiate the changes that accompany aging, the mind-body link becomes increasingly important.

Wall Pilates becomes a vehicle for self-discovery, allowing women to explore their physical skills and appreciate their bodies with gratitude.

Wall Pilates' wall support gives an added layer of stability, making it especially accessible to individuals over the age of 50.

This support enables a steady evolution of motions, resulting in a sensation of success.

Women create a robust attitude via persistent practice, understanding that strength is evaluated not just by external elements, but also by internal fortitude developed through conscious movement.

Furthermore, Wall Pilates' soft yet purposeful movements help to enhance flexibility and balance, which are important components of general well-being.

The coordination of breath and movement acts as a strong stress-relieving technique, helping women to face life's obstacles more easily.
As inner strength grows, a good ripple effect occurs in daily life, instilling a sense of empowerment and self-confidence.

Embracing mindful movements, particularly via disciplines such as Wall Pilates, enables women over 50 to gain inner strength.

The combination of purposeful movements, breath awareness, and wall support promotes a holistic approach to well-being, cultivating a resilient attitude that extends beyond the physical sphere.

This trip becomes a celebration of power, elegance, and the knowledge that comes from accepting one's own body and skills.

Chapter 5: specialized wall pilates for joint health

Specialized Wall Pilates provides a specialized approach to improving joint health, which is especially good for women over 50.

This one-of-a-kind exercise combines basic Pilates concepts with the support of a wall, resulting in a low-impact but extremely effective workout.

As women mature, joint health becomes a top priority. Specialized wall Pilates focuses on soft exercises that increase flexibility and strength while minimizing joint stress.

The wall acts as a stabilizing force, allowing participants to perform exercises that enhance their posture, balance, and total joint mobility.

This is critical for reducing the affects of aging since it targets regions prone to stiffness and pain.

The movements in Wall Pilates for Women Over 50 target particular muscle groups, improving core strength and balance.

This specific method, which emphasizes controlled motions and alignment, helps to reduce joint discomfort and avoid injuries.

The wall serves as a support structure, allowing participants to complete actions with confidence, making it a viable alternative for people of all fitness levels.

Wall Pilates promotes a comprehensive approach to wellbeing. It not only improves joint health but also increases mental well-being via mindful movement.

As women face the obstacles of aging, the mind-body connection developed by Wall

Pilates may be powerful, resulting in a higher overall quality of life.

Instructors that specialize in wall Pilates for women over 50 customize programs to meet specific needs, offering a personalized experience.

This approach's versatility makes it appropriate for those with joint issues or conditions, offering a safe and effective exercise alternative.

Specialized Wall Pilates for Women Over 50 is a deliberate and effective way to improve joint health.

Its emphasis on soft movements, wall support, and customized training distinguishes it as an accessible and empowering workout alternative for improving overall well-being.

Joint-Friendly Exercises

Wall Pilates, which is gentle on the joints and designed for ladies over 50, emerges as a comprehensive training program.

These joint-friendly exercises, which emphasize flexibility, strength, and balance, provide a revitalizing approach to training.

The wall acts as a stabilizing feature, providing a friendly atmosphere for those with varied levels of joint sensitivity.

Joint health becomes increasingly important for women as they become older. Wall Pilates offers a low-impact option that reduces joint stress while enhancing workout benefits.

Participants who engage in exercises that emphasize regulated muscular contractions get relief from joint soreness that is prevalent with high-impact activities.

The wall serves as a versatile prop, allowing for changes to accommodate varied fitness levels. This versatility is especially useful for women over 50, who may have variable degrees of mobility or joint difficulties.

The exercises include a variety of activities, from moderate stretches to focused muscle engagement, encouraging total joint mobility without putting the body under undue stress.

One of the primary benefits of Wall Pilates is its emphasis on core strength. Strengthening the core creates a sturdy foundation, easing the strain on joints during movement.

As women continue through the exercises, they not only increase joint flexibility, but also build a stronger, more robust musculature to support their overall health.

In addition to physical advantages, Wall Pilates promotes a mind-body connection.

The intentional and attentive execution of each action promotes mental concentration and relaxation, which aids in stress reduction, an important component of holistic health for women over 50.

Wall Pilates for women over 50 represents a harmonic combination of joint-friendly movements.

This training strategy creates a nurturing atmosphere by utilizing the wall's support, improving joint health, strength, and general well-being.

Addressing Arthritis and Joint Stiffness

Addressing arthritis and joint stiffness is critical, especially for women over 50, because these illnesses can greatly disrupt everyday living.

Wall Pilates is a mild yet effective way to improve joint flexibility and reduce pain.

As women get older, they are more likely to develop arthritis and joint stiffness. Wall Pilates, designed exclusively for this group, includes low-impact movements that emphasize joint mobility.Focusing on controlled motions reduces joint tension while increasing overall strength.

Wall Pilates might be especially good for women over 50 who suffer from arthritis because it focuses on joint-friendly motions. The integration of the wall adds support, making activities more accessible and reducing strain.

This strategy helps people improve their flexibility without increasing current joint problems.

The soft nature of Wall Pilates does not diminish its efficacy. Women can enhance their joint function by using a combination of stretching and strengthening activities.

The emphasis on perfect alignment ensures that motions are completed precisely, improving joint health and minimizing stiffness.

Furthermore, Wall Pilates promotes a mind-body connection and increases awareness of body mechanics. This awareness factor is critical for arthritis patients, as it allows them to modify their movements to their degree of comfort.

The comprehensive approach of Wall Pilates extends beyond physical advantages and contributes to general health.

Instructors that specialize in Wall Pilates for women over 50 customize classes to target particular arthritis and joint stiffness issues.

Customized routines take into account individual requirements and limits, resulting in a supportive atmosphere for women to recover control of their joint health.

Wall Pilates is a specialized solution for ladies over 50 dealing with arthritis and joint stiffness.

Its mild yet effective method develops joint flexibility, strength, and overall well-being, offering a comprehensive approach to addressing these typical age-related issues.

Adapting Pilates for Osteoporosis Prevention

Maintaining bone health becomes increasingly important as people age, especially for women over 50, who are more prone to osteoporosis.

Wall Pilates emerges as a useful workout strategy that is specifically suited to osteoporosis prevention.

This customized technique involves mild yet effective motions that address the unique requirements of those with weak bones.

Wall Pilates' emphasis on controlled, low-impact movements is consistent with osteoporosis prevention measures.

This type of Pilates promotes bone density by including weight-bearing movements in a healthy manner without putting individuals under undue pressure. The wall provides additional stability, lowering the chance of falls or fractures during the workout.

Wall Pilates for osteoporosis prevention combines spine-friendly routines while emphasizing postural alignment and core strength.

These exercises are designed to improve balance and coordination, both of which are important in minimizing the probability of falls, which are a major worry for people with osteoporosis.

The wall serves as a prop for support during workouts such as leg lifts and side stretches, guaranteeing good form while maintaining safety.

Wall Pilates enhances flexibility and joint mobility, which helps to alleviate stiffness linked with aging and osteoporosis. The controlled stretches in the program improve range of motion while reducing stress on sensitive regions. This comprehensive method not only improves bones but also promotes general health.

Adapting Pilates for osteoporosis prevention via Wall Pilates offers a personalized solution for women over 50, encouraging bone health without the need for excessive repetition of high-impact exercises.

With its emphasis on regulated movements, stability, and flexibility, Wall Pilates emerges as a thoughtful and practical technique for maintaining skeletal health in older people.

Chapter 6: Holistic Wellness Integration

Holistic wellness integration for women over 50 goes beyond traditional workout routines, embracing a holistic health strategy based on Wall Pilates principles.

This mindful practice emphasizes not just physical strength but also mental and emotional well-being, cultivating a harmonious connection between mind, body, and spirit.

Wall Pilates for women over 50 is a unique adaptation of basic Pilates exercises that takes advantage of a wall's support, increasing stability and safety.

This combination of Pilates with a vertical aspect converts the workout into a whole experience that targets core strength, balance, and flexibility. The mild yet powerful exercises address the unique requirements of elderly women, boosting their total health and energy.

Integrating holistic wellness ideas into Wall Pilates requires a holistic perspective. It facilitates attentive breathing methods, which reduce stress and improve mental clarity.

Women over 50 can increase their lung capacity by integrating these breathing routines with Pilates exercises, which promote respiratory health and general vitality.

Furthermore, Wall Pilates promotes awareness of body alignment, which aids in better posture and less joint strain. This integrated strategy helps to avoid injuries while also addressing common aging problems like osteoporosis and joint stiffness. The emphasis on regulated movements matches the body's natural rhythms, making it an excellent choice for ladies looking for a long-lasting and pleasurable workout regimen.

Beyond the physical components, comprehensive integration promotes emotional resilience. Wall Pilates promotes self-reflection and mindfulness, which has a favorable effect on mental health.

This mind-body connection is especially advantageous for women dealing with the challenges and changes that come with aging, as it promotes a sense of empowerment and wellbeing.

Holistic Wellness Integration with Wall Pilates for women over 50 provides a transforming experience that goes beyond fitness. It evolves into a comprehensive lifestyle approach that benefits not just the body, but also the mind and soul, paving the way for long-term well-being.

Nutrition Tips for Women over 50

As women get older, eating a balanced diet becomes increasingly important for their general health.

Nutritional demands change with age, affecting energy levels, bone health, and illness prevention.

Here are thorough and concise nutrition suggestions suited for women in this age group:

1. Prioritize. Calcium and Vitamin D: Aging bones demand special care. Consume enough amounts of calcium-rich foods such as dairy, leafy greens, and fortified goods. Combine this with vitamin D sources like fatty fish and sun exposure to improve calcium absorption.

2. Protein-Rich Diet: A sufficient protein intake promotes muscular mass, which tends to decline with age. To achieve protein requirements, consume lean meats, poultry, fish, eggs, dairy products, legumes, and nuts.

3. *Fiber for Digestive Health:* Eat fiber-rich foods such as whole grains, fruits, vegetables, and legumes to improve digestive health and weight management. Fiber also helps to avoid constipation, a typical issue in this age range.

4. *Hydration Matters:* Dehydration risks increase with age, affecting skin health and general physical processes. Ensure an appropriate water intake and include hydrating meals like water-rich fruits and vegetables.

5. *Omega-3 Fatty Acids:* Consume omega-3-rich foods such as fatty fish (salmon, mackerel), flaxseeds, and walnuts to improve heart health and cognitive performance.

6. *Limit salt and Processed Foods:* To control blood pressure, reduce salt consumption. To reduce salt levels, eat less processed and packaged meals and more fresh, natural foods.

7. *Adequate Iron Intake:* After menopause, women's iron needs drop. To improve iron absorption, eat iron-rich plant foods such beans, lentils, and fortified cereals while also getting enough vitamin C.

8. *Keep an eye on Vitamin B12 and Folate levels:* As we age, our ability to absorb nutrients changes. To promote energy metabolism and red blood cell synthesis, consume B12 (fish, dairy, fortified cereals) and folate (leafy greens, citrus fruits) on a regular basis.

9. *Monitor Caloric Intake:* As we age, our metabolic rate lowers, making weight control difficult. Calorie consumption should be adjusted based on activity level, with the goal of achieving a well-balanced diet that is rich in nutrients.

10. *Consult a Healthcare Professional:* Individual health problems and medications might have an influence on dietary requirements.
Consult with healthcare specialists on a regular basis to customize dietary suggestions for your specific health needs.

Women over 50 may improve their health and live a more happy life by following these eating guidelines.

Sleep and Recovery Strategies

Quality sleep and good recovery mechanisms are critical to improving overall well-being, particularly for women over 50 who participate in Wall Pilates.

Restorative sleep becomes increasingly important as the body matures. Sleep allows the body to heal and rejuvenate, which helps with muscular recovery and cognitive function.

For women adopting Wall Pilates into their regimen, getting enough sleep is critical to enjoying the full advantages of this low-impact, strengthening exercise.

To improve sleep quality, a consistent sleep pattern is required. Creating a soothing pre-bedtime routine and making the sleep environment pleasant all contribute to a good night's sleep. Techniques like mindfulness meditation can be very effective for relaxing.

In addition, focused recuperation measures are essential for women over 50 who do Wall Pilates.

This involves enough water to maintain joint function and muscle flexibility. Hydration helps to flush out toxins and improves nutrition delivery, therefore helping the body's healing processes.

Nutrition is also very important. A well-balanced diet high in protein, antioxidants, and anti-inflammatory foods promotes muscle recovery and lowers inflammation, which enhances the effects of Wall Pilates.

 Consider visiting a nutritionist to adapt your food choices to your specific needs.

Active rehabilitation, which includes light workouts or activities such as walking or swimming, can help relieve muscular discomfort caused by Pilates. Furthermore, combining flexibility exercises improves joint mobility while decreasing the chance of injury.

Stress management is essential for general well-being. Activities that encourage relaxation, such as deep breathing exercises or mild yoga, can help reduce stress and improve sleep and recuperation.

Women over 50 may maximize the advantages of Wall Pilates by including these sleep and recovery practices into their daily routines, promoting a holistic approach to health and longevity.

Creating a holistic lifestyle within wall pilates

Wall Pilates can help women over 50 live a more complete lifestyle. This low-impact workout regimen not only builds physical strength but also promotes mental well-being, making it an excellent alternative for individuals looking for a holistic approach to health.

Wall Pilates focuses on core strength, flexibility, and balance, all of which are important for women in their fifties who want to be healthy in general.

The wall's support gives an added layer of stability, lowering the chance of harm and allowing people to focus on controlled motions. This tailored workout encourages lean muscle growth, which helps women maintain a healthy weight and supports bone density, both of which are important factors for women of this age.

Beyond the physical benefits, Wall Pilates has a significant impact on mental wellness.

The attentive breathing and attention necessary for the exercise help to reduce stress and promote mental clarity.

As women manage the difficulties of life beyond 50, the mind-body link becomes a vital tool for dealing with everyday challenges and maintaining a happy attitude.

Furthermore, including Wall Pilates into a regular regimen promotes discipline and consistency.

Consistent practice not only improves physical fitness, but it also provides a sense of accomplishment and raises self-esteem. This comprehensive strategy goes beyond the workout itself, impacting food choices, sleep patterns, and general lifestyle behaviors.

Building a holistic lifestyle around Wall Pilates entails incorporating it into a larger self-care framework.

This might involve eating a well-balanced and healthy diet, staying hydrated, and adding other thoughtful activities like meditation or taking regular nature walks.

The combination of these aspects promotes a complete approach to health and well-being that addresses the special requirements of women over 50, resulting in increased lifespan and vitality.

Embracing Wall Pilates as an integral part of a holistic lifestyle for women over 50 provides a comprehensive approach to wellness. This mindful exercise strategy not only improves the body but also promotes mental resilience, laying the groundwork for

total well-being as people gracefully traverse
the second half of their lives.

Chapter 7: Progression and Longevity in Wall Pilates Practices

In the world of fitness, Wall Pilates emerges as a revolutionary technique, particularly for women over 50 looking to advance and sustain their wellness journey.

This low-impact training strategy emphasizes core strength, flexibility, and balance while using a vertical surface for support. As people age, preserving these fundamental qualities becomes increasingly important for their general well-being.

Women over 50 progress through Wall Pilates by gradually increasing the difficulty and intensity. Beginning with basic exercises that emphasize stability, practitioners progress to increasingly difficult motions. The vertical alignment against the wall increases posture awareness, promotes spinal health, and reduces the effects of aging on the skeletal structure.

This development guarantees a personalized approach, allowing people to modify the exercise to their own fitness levels and physical ailments.

The longevity of the wall Pilates is based on adaptation and sustainability. The exercises' moderate nature decreases joint tension, making them an excellent alternative for anyone dealing with the aging process.

The wall provides an added layer of support, giving practitioners confidence as they explore their range of motion.

Consistent practice increases muscular endurance and resilience, which contributes to long-term functional fitness.

Wall Pilates tackles special problems for women over the age of 50, including bone density and joint health.

The regulated motions activate deep muscles, increasing overall strength without putting unnecessary strain on the body.

This emphasis on holistic wellbeing goes beyond the physical to include mental and emotional advantages.

Wall Pilates cultivates the mind-body connection, which improves cognitive function and decreases stress, leading to overall wellness.

Wall Pilates provides a creative route for women over 50 to grow and maintain their health.
Its personalized approach, emphasis on core strength, and mild yet powerful techniques make it an excellent practice for boosting total well-being as people age gracefully.

Gradual Progression Guidelines

Guiding women over 50 through the progressive development of Wall Pilates requires a deliberate approach that promotes safety and efficacy.

Begin with easy warm-up activities to get the body ready for the workout. Concentrate on regulated breathing to promote relaxation and calm the mind.

Use basic motions like pelvic tilts and mild stretches to improve flexibility and joint mobility.

As the session progresses, incorporate low-impact movements that target particular muscle groups while focusing the core and staying connected to the breath.

Include the use of a stability ball to give variation and challenge while developing balance. Increase the difficulty level of movements gradually, taking into account individual capacities.

Transition to wall. Pilates movements that use the assistance of a wall for stability. Wall squats and leg lifts work the lower body, increasing strength and endurance. Integrate exercises such as wall planks to enhance core stability and posture.

Stress the significance of perfect form in preventing strain and lowering the chance of injury.

Incorporate resistance training using resistance bands or modest weights to gradually increase physical strength. Concentrate on complex motions that work numerous muscular groups at once.

This comprehensive strategy promotes general fitness and combats age-related muscle loss.

As the program comes to an end, lead participants through a series of relaxing stretches and activities.

Emphasize the significance of listening to their body and making changes as necessary.
Encourage frequent practice, with an emphasis on consistency over intensity.

Individual requirements and talents should be considered while designing the path, since each woman may have distinct obstacles and ambitions.

Make accommodations for people with special problems, such as joint pain or limited mobility.

The aim on empowering women over 50 via progressive Wall Pilates growth is to cultivate a pleasant and sustainable fitness path that leads to overall well-being.

Adapting workouts for long-term sustainability

Long-term sustainability in exercises is critical, especially for women over 50 who participate in Wall Pilates.

This low-impact workout is known for improving flexibility, strength, and posture, making it an excellent choice for anyone seeking long-term fitness benefits.

To modify workouts for long-term success, focus on incremental alterations. Begin with basic exercises and progressively increase the intensity as your strength and endurance develop.

Including a diversity of motions reduces boredom and keeps the body engaged, ensuring ongoing improvement while avoiding burnout or injury.

Workouts should be tailored to each individual's needs. Women over 50 may have different exercise levels and health concerns.

Customizing exercises based on personal talents and constraints promotes a better fitness experience. Make adaptations to suit any current ailments or joint sensitivities, guaranteeing a safe and pleasurable workout.

Incorporating mindfulness into Wall Pilates improves the mind-body connection. During workouts, concentrate and use good breathing methods.

This not only increases the efficacy of each action, but it also promotes relaxation, reduces tension, and improves general well-being.

Long-term success relies heavily on consistency. Create a simple and realistic fitness regimen that works with your everyday habits. Establishing a habit instills a sense of dedication, making it simpler to stick to the workout plan over time. Celebrate modest accomplishments to reinforce positive habits and drive.

Pay attention to the body's signals and change workouts accordingly. Periodic revision of fitness objectives, as well as altering routines to meet changing demands, promotes ongoing growth and avoids plateaus.

Adapting Wall Pilates programs for women over 50 entails progressive growth, customisation, mindfulness, consistency, and constant self-evaluation.

By adhering to these principles, people may develop a long-term workout program that promotes longevity and well-being.

Celebrating Achievements and Milestones

Accepting successes and milestones is a critical component of human development and well-being. For women over 50, the path of celebrating milestones takes on a special meaning, and Wall Pilates becomes an invaluable ally in this endeavors.

When women reach the age of 50, they frequently enter a period of transition in their lives.

Among the modifications, including wall Pilates into their practice delivers not only physical advantages but also acts as a sign of tenacity and drive

The exercise not only improves strength and flexibility, but it also provides a sense of success when progress is achieved.

The growing mastery of difficult exercises is an important part of the Wall Pilates milestone celebrations.

Every effective execution of a posture or longer time in a stance is a victory worth celebrating. These wins foster a positive mentality and promote the notion that aging is no obstacle to accomplishing new goals.

Furthermore, the social component of Wall Pilates sessions creates a friendly environment for women over 50 to discuss and celebrate their accomplishments.

The camaraderie developed during these sessions builds a feeling of community and reciprocal support, transforming individual achievements into shared joys.

Celebrating Milestones in Wall Pilates is about more than just physical capability; it's about understanding the mental and emotional strength that comes from persistent practice. As women overcome new hurdles, they develop a mentality that goes beyond the studio, positively impacting many aspects of their lives.

In essence, celebrating accomplishments and milestones in Wall Pilates for women over 50 is a comprehensive experience.

It demonstrates the force of dedication, the joy of shared triumphs, and the tremendous influence of adopting a healthy and active lifestyle as a basis for future success.

CONCLUSION

Wall Pilates emerges as a comprehensive and transformational exercise method designed exclusively for ladies over 50.

This low-impact exercise strategy serves this demographic's specific physical and emotional demands, boosting total well-being.

Wall Pilates promotes increased flexibility, core strength, and posture by combining regulated movements, breathing methods, and conscious attention.

The use of the wall in Pilates for women over 50 acts as a stabilizing factor, lowering the danger of strain and damage.

This adaptation addresses age-related reductions in muscle mass and bone density,

resulting in a safer and more sustainable training plan.
Furthermore, wall Pilates promotes pelvic floor activation, which is essential for women of this age to preserve bladder control and pelvic health.

Wall Pilates provides substantial mental involvement, fostering mindfulness and stress reduction in addition to its physical advantages.

The purposeful concentration on breathing and precise movements fosters a mind-body connection, which helps to promote mental clarity and emotional well-being.

As women move through the numerous exercises, they not only improve their physical fitness but also feel empowered and accomplished.

Wall Pilates for women over 50 is a holistic wellness solution that addresses the demographic's specific difficulties and ambitions. By combining targeted workouts, thoughtful practices, and adaptability, it promotes a meaningful and long-term approach to fitness, encouraging health and vitality throughout the latter half of life.

Workout planner to help you record your progress.

Workout PLANNER

Week ______________________ Month ______________________

	WORKOUT	MEALS	GOALS
Monday			
Tuesday			
Wednesday			
Thursday			
Friday			
Saturday			
Sunday			

Workout PLANNER

Week _______________________   Month _______________________

	WORKOUT	MEALS	GOALS
Monday			

	WORKOUT	MEALS	GOALS
Tuesday			

	WORKOUT	MEALS	GOALS
Wednesday			

	WORKOUT	MEALS	GOALS
Thursday			

	WORKOUT	MEALS	GOALS
Friday			

	WORKOUT	MEALS	GOALS
Saturday			

	WORKOUT	MEALS	GOALS
Sunday			

Workout PLANNER

Week _______________   Month _______________

	WORKOUT	MEALS	GOALS
Monday			
Tuesday			
Wednesday			
Thursday			
Friday			
Saturday			
Sunday			

Workout PLANNER

Week .... *Month* ....

	WORKOUT	MEALS	GOALS
Monday			

	WORKOUT	MEALS	GOALS
Tuesday			

	WORKOUT	MEALS	GOALS
Wednesday			

	WORKOUT	MEALS	GOALS
Thursday			

	WORKOUT	MEALS	GOALS
Friday			

	WORKOUT	MEALS	GOALS
Saturday			

	WORKOUT	MEALS	GOALS
Sunday			

Workout PLANNER

Week _______________   Month _______________

Monday

WORKOUT	MEALS	GOALS

Tuesday

WORKOUT	MEALS	GOALS

Wednesday

WORKOUT	MEALS	GOALS

Thursday

WORKOUT	MEALS	GOALS

Friday

WORKOUT	MEALS	GOALS

Saturday

WORKOUT	MEALS	GOALS

Sunday

WORKOUT	MEALS	GOALS

Workout PLANNER

Week .... *Month* ....

Monday	WORKOUT	MEALS	GOALS

Tuesday	WORKOUT	MEALS	GOALS

Wednesday	WORKOUT	MEALS	GOALS

Thursday	WORKOUT		GOALS

Friday	WORKOUT	MEALS	GOALS

Saturday	WORKOUT	MEALS	GOALS

Sunday	WORKOUT	MEALS	GOALS

Workout PLANNER

Week _______________________   Month _______________________

	WORKOUT	MEALS	GOALS
Monday			

	WORKOUT	MEALS	GOALS
Tuesday			

	WORKOUT	MEALS	GOALS
Wednesday			

	WORKOUT	MEALS	GOALS
Thursday			

	WORKOUT	MEALS	GOALS
Friday			

	WORKOUT	MEALS	GOALS
Saturday			

	WORKOUT	MEALS	GOALS
Sunday			

Workout PLANNER

Week ____________________   Month ____________________

	WORKOUT	MEALS	GOALS
Monday			
Tuesday			
Wednesday			
Thursday			
Friday			
Saturday			
Sunday			

Week _______________________ Month _______________________

	WORKOUT	MEALS	GOALS
Monday			

	WORKOUT	MEALS	GOALS
Tuesday			

	WORKOUT	MEALS	GOALS
Wednesday			

	WORKOUT		GOALS
Thursday			

	WORKOUT	MEALS	GOALS
Friday			

	WORKOUT	MEALS	GOALS
Saturday			

	WORKOUT	MEALS	GOALS
Sunday			

Workout *PLANNER*

Week .... *Month* ....

	WORKOUT	MEALS	GOALS
Monday			

	WORKOUT	MEALS	GOALS
Tuesday			

	WORKOUT	MEALS	GOALS
Wednesday			

	WORKOUT		GOALS
Thursday			

	WORKOUT	MEALS	GOALS
Friday			

	WORKOUT	MEALS	GOALS
Saturday			

	WORKOUT	MEALS	GOALS
Sunday			

Workout PLANNER

Week .... *Month* ....

Monday	WORKOUT	MEALS	GOALS

Tuesday	WORKOUT	MEALS	GOALS

Wednesday	WORKOUT	MEALS	GOALS

Thursday	WORKOUT		GOALS

Friday	WORKOUT	MEALS	GOALS

Saturday	WORKOUT	MEALS	GOALS

Sunday	WORKOUT	MEALS	GOALS

Workout PLANNER

Week .... Month ....

	WORKOUT	MEALS	GOALS
Monday			
Tuesday			
Wednesday			
Thursday			
Friday			
Saturday			
Sunday			

Workout PLANNER

Week .... *Month* ....

	WORKOUT	MEALS	GOALS
Monday			

	WORKOUT	MEALS	GOALS
Tuesday			

	WORKOUT	MEALS	GOALS
Wednesday			

	WORKOUT		GOALS
Thursday			

	WORKOUT	MEALS	GOALS
Friday			

	WORKOUT	MEALS	GOALS
Saturday			

	WORKOUT	MEALS	GOALS
Sunday			

Workout PLANNER

Week .... Month ....

	WORKOUT	MEALS	GOALS
Monday			

	WORKOUT	MEALS	GOALS
Tuesday			

	WORKOUT	MEALS	GOALS
Wednesday			

	WORKOUT		GOALS
Thursday			

	WORKOUT	MEALS	GOALS
Friday			

	WORKOUT	MEALS	GOALS
Saturday			

	WORKOUT	MEALS	GOALS
Sunday			

Workout PLANNER

Week ____________________   Month ____________________

Monday	WORKOUT	MEALS	GOALS

Tuesday	WORKOUT	MEALS	GOALS

Wednesday	WORKOUT	MEALS	GOALS

Thursday	WORKOUT		GOALS

Friday	WORKOUT	MEALS	GOALS

Saturday	WORKOUT	MEALS	GOALS

Sunday	WORKOUT	MEALS	GOALS

Workout PLANNER

Week ___________________ Month ___________________

	WORKOUT	MEALS	GOALS
Monday			

	WORKOUT	MEALS	GOALS
Tuesday			

	WORKOUT	MEALS	GOALS
Wednesday			

	WORKOUT	MEALS	GOALS
Thursday			

	WORKOUT	MEALS	GOALS
Friday			

	WORKOUT	MEALS	GOALS
Saturday			

	WORKOUT	MEALS	GOALS
Sunday			

Workout PLANNER

Week ....   Month ....

	WORKOUT	MEALS	GOALS
Monday			

	WORKOUT	MEALS	GOALS
Tuesday			

	WORKOUT	MEALS	GOALS
Wednesday			

	WORKOUT		GOALS
Thursday			

	WORKOUT	MEALS	GOALS
Friday			

	WORKOUT	MEALS	GOALS
Saturday			

	WORKOUT	MEALS	GOALS
Sunday			

Workout PLANNER

Week .... Month ....

	WORKOUT	MEALS	GOALS
Monday			

	WORKOUT	MEALS	GOALS
Tuesday			

	WORKOUT	MEALS	GOALS
Wednesday			

	WORKOUT		GOALS
Thursday			

	WORKOUT	MEALS	GOALS
Friday			

	WORKOUT	MEALS	GOALS
Saturday			

	WORKOUT	MEALS	GOALS
Sunday			

Workout PLANNER

Week .... *Month* ....

	WORKOUT	MEALS	GOALS
Monday			

	WORKOUT	MEALS	GOALS
Tuesday			

	WORKOUT	MEALS	GOALS
Wednesday			

	WORKOUT		GOALS
Thursday			

	WORKOUT	MEALS	GOALS
Friday			

	WORKOUT	MEALS	GOALS
Saturday			

	WORKOUT	MEALS	GOALS
Sunday			

Workout PLANNER

Week ....   Month ....

Monday	WORKOUT	MEALS	GOALS

Tuesday	WORKOUT	MEALS	GOALS

Wednesday	WORKOUT	MEALS	GOALS

Thursday	WORKOUT	MEALS	GOALS

Friday	WORKOUT	MEALS	GOALS

Saturday	WORKOUT	MEALS	GOALS

Sunday	WORKOUT	MEALS	GOALS

Workout PLANNER

Week .... *Month* ....

Monday	WORKOUT	MEALS	GOALS

Tuesday	WORKOUT	MEALS	GOALS

Wednesday	WORKOUT	MEALS	GOALS

Thursday	WORKOUT		GOALS

Friday	WORKOUT	MEALS	GOALS

Saturday	WORKOUT	MEALS	GOALS

Sunday	WORKOUT	MEALS	GOALS

Workout PLANNER

Week .... Month ....

	WORKOUT	MEALS	GOALS
Monday			

	WORKOUT	MEALS	GOALS
Tuesday			

	WORKOUT	MEALS	GOALS
Wednesday			

	WORKOUT	MEALS	GOALS
Thursday			

	WORKOUT	MEALS	GOALS
Friday			

	WORKOUT	MEALS	GOALS
Saturday			

	WORKOUT	MEALS	GOALS
Sunday			

Workout PLANNER

Week ________________ Month ________________

	WORKOUT	MEALS	GOALS
Monday			

	WORKOUT	MEALS	GOALS
Tuesday			

	WORKOUT	MEALS	GOALS
Wednesday			

	WORKOUT	MEALS	GOALS
Thursday			

	WORKOUT	MEALS	GOALS
Friday			

	WORKOUT	MEALS	GOALS
Saturday			

	WORKOUT	MEALS	GOALS
Sunday			

Workout PLANNER

Week .... Month ....

	WORKOUT	MEALS	GOALS
Monday			

	WORKOUT	MEALS	GOALS
Tuesday			

	WORKOUT	MEALS	GOALS
Wednesday			

	WORKOUT		GOALS
Thursday			

	WORKOUT	MEALS	GOALS
Friday			

	WORKOUT	MEALS	GOALS
Saturday			

	WORKOUT	MEALS	GOALS
Sunday			

Workout PLANNER

Week .... Month ....

Monday	WORKOUT	MEALS	GOALS

Tuesday	WORKOUT	MEALS	GOALS

Wednesday	WORKOUT	MEALS	GOALS

Thursday	WORKOUT		GOALS

Friday	WORKOUT	MEALS	GOALS

Saturday	WORKOUT	MEALS	GOALS

Sunday	WORKOUT	MEALS	GOALS

Workout PLANNER

Week .... Month ....

Monday

WORKOUT	MEALS	GOALS

Tuesday

WORKOUT	MEALS	GOALS

Wednesday

WORKOUT	MEALS	GOALS

Thursday

WORKOUT		GOALS

Friday

WORKOUT	MEALS	GOALS

Saturday

WORKOUT	MEALS	GOALS

Sunday

WORKOUT	MEALS	GOALS

Workout PLANNER

Week ______________________   Month ______________________

	WORKOUT	MEALS	GOALS
Monday			

	WORKOUT	MEALS	GOALS
Tuesday			

	WORKOUT	MEALS	GOALS
Wednesday			

	WORKOUT		GOALS
Thursday			

	WORKOUT	MEALS	GOALS
Friday			

	WORKOUT	MEALS	GOALS
Saturday			

	WORKOUT	MEALS	GOALS
Sunday			

Workout PLANNER

Week _______________ Month _______________

Monday	WORKOUT	MEALS	GOALS

Tuesday	WORKOUT	MEALS	GOALS

Wednesday	WORKOUT	MEALS	GOALS

Thursday	WORKOUT		GOALS

Friday	WORKOUT	MEALS	GOALS

Saturday	WORKOUT	MEALS	GOALS

Sunday	WORKOUT	MEALS	GOALS

Workout PLANNER

Week .... Month ....

Monday	WORKOUT	MEALS	GOALS

Tuesday	WORKOUT	MEALS	GOALS

Wednesday	WORKOUT	MEALS	GOALS

Thursday	WORKOUT		GOALS

Friday	WORKOUT	MEALS	GOALS

Saturday	WORKOUT	MEALS	GOALS

Sunday	WORKOUT	MEALS	GOALS

Week _______________________   Month _______________________

	WORKOUT	MEALS	GOALS
Monday			

	WORKOUT	MEALS	GOALS
Tuesday			

	WORKOUT	MEALS	GOALS
Wednesday			

	WORKOUT		GOALS
Thursday			

	WORKOUT	MEALS	GOALS
Friday			

	WORKOUT	MEALS	GOALS
Saturday			

	WORKOUT	MEALS	GOALS
Sunday			

Workout PLANNER

Week .... *Month* ....

	WORKOUT	MEALS	GOALS
Monday			

	WORKOUT	MEALS	GOALS
Tuesday			

	WORKOUT	MEALS	GOALS
Wednesday			

	WORKOUT	MEALS	GOALS
Thursday			

	WORKOUT	MEALS	GOALS
Friday			

	WORKOUT	MEALS	GOALS
Saturday			

	WORKOUT	MEALS	GOALS
Sunday			

Workout PLANNER

Week ....   Month ....

	WORKOUT	MEALS	GOALS
Monday			

	WORKOUT	MEALS	GOALS
Tuesday			

	WORKOUT	MEALS	GOALS
Wednesday			

	WORKOUT		GOALS
Thursday			

	WORKOUT	MEALS	GOALS
Friday			

	WORKOUT	MEALS	GOALS
Saturday			

	WORKOUT	MEALS	GOALS
Sunday			

Workout PLANNER

Week.. Month....................

Monday	WORKOUT	MEALS	GOALS

Tuesday	WORKOUT	MEALS	GOALS

Wednesday	WORKOUT	MEALS	GOALS

Thursday	WORKOUT		GOALS

Friday	WORKOUT	MEALS	GOALS

Saturday	WORKOUT	MEALS	GOALS

Sunday	WORKOUT	MEALS	GOALS

Workout PLANNER

Week .... Month ....

Monday	WORKOUT	MEALS	GOALS

Tuesday	WORKOUT	MEALS	GOALS

Wednesday	WORKOUT	MEALS	GOALS

Thursday	WORKOUT		GOALS

Friday	WORKOUT	MEALS	GOALS

Saturday	WORKOUT	MEALS	GOALS

Sunday	WORKOUT	MEALS	GOALS

Workout PLANNER

Week .... Month ....

	WORKOUT	MEALS	GOALS
Monday			

	WORKOUT	MEALS	GOALS
Tuesday			

	WORKOUT	MEALS	GOALS
Wednesday			

	WORKOUT	MEALS	GOALS
Thursday			

	WORKOUT	MEALS	GOALS
Friday			

	WORKOUT	MEALS	GOALS
Saturday			

	WORKOUT	MEALS	GOALS
Sunday			

Workout PLANNER

Week _______________   Month _______________

	WORKOUT	MEALS	GOALS
Monday			

	WORKOUT	MEALS	GOALS
Tuesday			

	WORKOUT	MEALS	GOALS
Wednesday			

	WORKOUT		GOALS
Thursday			

	WORKOUT	MEALS	GOALS
Friday			

	WORKOUT	MEALS	GOALS
Saturday			

	WORKOUT	MEALS	GOALS
Sunday			

Workout PLANNER

Week .... *Month* ....

	WORKOUT	MEALS	GOALS
Monday			

	WORKOUT	MEALS	GOALS
Tuesday			

	WORKOUT	MEALS	GOALS
Wednesday			

	WORKOUT	MEALS	GOALS
Thursday			

	WORKOUT	MEALS	GOALS
Friday			

	WORKOUT	MEALS	GOALS
Saturday			

	WORKOUT	MEALS	GOALS
Sunday			

Workout PLANNER

Week .... Month ....

	WORKOUT	MEALS	GOALS
Monday			

	WORKOUT	MEALS	GOALS
Tuesday			

	WORKOUT	MEALS	GOALS
Wednesday			

	WORKOUT		GOALS
Thursday			

	WORKOUT	MEALS	GOALS
Friday			

	WORKOUT	MEALS	GOALS
Saturday			

	WORKOUT	MEALS	GOALS
Sunday			

Workout PLANNER

Week ....   *Month* ....

	WORKOUT	MEALS	GOALS
Monday			

	WORKOUT	MEALS	GOALS
Tuesday			

	WORKOUT	MEALS	GOALS
Wednesday			

	WORKOUT		GOALS
Thursday			

	WORKOUT	MEALS	GOALS
Friday			

	WORKOUT	MEALS	GOALS
Saturday			

	WORKOUT	MEALS	GOALS
Sunday			

Workout PLANNER

Week _____________ Month _____________

Monday	WORKOUT	MEALS	GOALS

Tuesday	WORKOUT	MEALS	GOALS

Wednesday	WORKOUT	MEALS	GOALS

Thursday	WORKOUT		GOALS

Friday	WORKOUT	MEALS	GOALS

Saturday	WORKOUT	MEALS	GOALS

Sunday	WORKOUT	MEALS	GOALS

Workout PLANNER

Week .... *Month* ....

	WORKOUT	MEALS	GOALS
Monday			

	WORKOUT	MEALS	GOALS
Tuesday			

	WORKOUT	MEALS	GOALS
Wednesday			

	WORKOUT		GOALS
Thursday			

	WORKOUT	MEALS	GOALS
Friday			

	WORKOUT	MEALS	GOALS
Saturday			

	WORKOUT	MEALS	GOALS
Sunday			

Workout PLANNER

Week ________________   Month ________________

Monday	WORKOUT	MEALS	GOALS

Tuesday	WORKOUT	MEALS	GOALS

Wednesday	WORKOUT	MEALS	GOALS

Thursday	WORKOUT		GOALS

Friday	WORKOUT	MEALS	GOALS

Saturday	WORKOUT	MEALS	GOALS

Sunday	WORKOUT	MEALS	GOALS

Workout PLANNER

Week _______________________ Month _______________________

	WORKOUT	MEALS	GOALS
Monday			
Tuesday			
Wednesday			
Thursday			
Friday			
Saturday			
Sunday			

Workout PLANNER

Week .... Month ....

	WORKOUT	MEALS	GOALS
Monday			

	WORKOUT	MEALS	GOALS
Tuesday			

	WORKOUT	MEALS	GOALS
Wednesday			

	WORKOUT		GOALS
Thursday			

	WORKOUT	MEALS	GOALS
Friday			

	WORKOUT	MEALS	GOALS
Saturday			

	WORKOUT	MEALS	GOALS
Sunday			

Workout PLANNER

Week ____________________   Month ____________________

	WORKOUT	MEALS	GOALS
Monday			

	WORKOUT	MEALS	GOALS
Tuesday			

	WORKOUT	MEALS	GOALS
Wednesday			

	WORKOUT		GOALS
Thursday			

	WORKOUT	MEALS	GOALS
Friday			

	WORKOUT	MEALS	GOALS
Saturday			

	WORKOUT	MEALS	GOALS
Sunday			

Workout PLANNER

Week .... Month ....

	WORKOUT	MEALS	GOALS
Monday			

	WORKOUT	MEALS	GOALS
Tuesday			

	WORKOUT	MEALS	GOALS
Wednesday			

	WORKOUT	MEALS	GOALS
Thursday			

	WORKOUT	MEALS	GOALS
Friday			

	WORKOUT	MEALS	GOALS
Saturday			

	WORKOUT	MEALS	GOALS
Sunday			

Workout PLANNER

Week .... Month ....

	WORKOUT	MEALS	GOALS
Monday			

	WORKOUT	MEALS	GOALS
Tuesday			

	WORKOUT	MEALS	GOALS
Wednesday			

	WORKOUT		GOALS
Thursday			

	WORKOUT	MEALS	GOALS
Friday			

	WORKOUT	MEALS	GOALS
Saturday			

	WORKOUT	MEALS	GOALS
Sunday			

Workout PLANNER

Week .... *Month* ....

Monday	WORKOUT	MEALS	GOALS

Tuesday	WORKOUT	MEALS	GOALS

Wednesday	WORKOUT	MEALS	GOALS

Thursday	WORKOUT		GOALS

Friday	WORKOUT	MEALS	GOALS

Saturday	WORKOUT	MEALS	GOALS

Sunday	WORKOUT	MEALS	GOALS

Workout PLANNER

Week .... *Month* ....

	WORKOUT	MEALS	GOALS
Monday			

	WORKOUT	MEALS	GOALS
Tuesday			

	WORKOUT	MEALS	GOALS
Wednesday			

	WORKOUT		GOALS
Thursday			

	WORKOUT	MEALS	GOALS
Friday			

	WORKOUT	MEALS	GOALS
Saturday			

	WORKOUT	MEALS	GOALS
Sunday			

Week .... Month ....

	WORKOUT	MEALS	GOALS
Monday			

	WORKOUT	MEALS	GOALS
Tuesday			

	WORKOUT	MEALS	GOALS
Wednesday			

	WORKOUT	MEALS	GOALS
Thursday			

	WORKOUT	MEALS	GOALS
Friday			

	WORKOUT	MEALS	GOALS
Saturday			

	WORKOUT	MEALS	GOALS
Sunday			

Workout PLANNER

Week _______________ *Month* _______________

Monday	WORKOUT	MEALS	GOALS

Tuesday	WORKOUT	MEALS	GOALS

Wednesday	WORKOUT	MEALS	GOALS

Thursday	WORKOUT		GOALS

Friday	WORKOUT	MEALS	GOALS

Saturday	WORKOUT	MEALS	GOALS

Sunday	WORKOUT	MEALS	GOALS

Workout PLANNER

Week .... Month ....

	WORKOUT	MEALS	GOALS
Monday			

	WORKOUT	MEALS	GOALS
Tuesday			

	WORKOUT	MEALS	GOALS
Wednesday			

	WORKOUT	MEALS	GOALS
Thursday			

	WORKOUT	MEALS	GOALS
Friday			

	WORKOUT	MEALS	GOALS
Saturday			

	WORKOUT	MEALS	GOALS
Sunday			

Workout PLANNER

Week .... Month ....

	WORKOUT	MEALS	GOALS
Monday			

	WORKOUT	MEALS	GOALS
Tuesday			

	WORKOUT	MEALS	GOALS
Wednesday			

	WORKOUT		GOALS
Thursday			

	WORKOUT	MEALS	GOALS
Friday			

	WORKOUT	MEALS	GOALS
Saturday			

	WORKOUT	MEALS	GOALS
Sunday			

Workout PLANNER

Week _______________   Month _______________

Monday	WORKOUT	MEALS	GOALS

Tuesday	WORKOUT	MEALS	GOALS

Wednesday	WORKOUT	MEALS	GOALS

Thursday	WORKOUT		GOALS

Friday	WORKOUT	MEALS	GOALS

Saturday	WORKOUT	MEALS	GOALS

Sunday	WORKOUT	MEALS	GOALS

Workout PLANNER

Week ___________ Month ___________

Monday

WORKOUT	MEALS	GOALS

Tuesday

WORKOUT	MEALS	GOALS

Wednesday

WORKOUT	MEALS	GOALS

Thursday

WORKOUT		GOALS

Friday

WORKOUT	MEALS	GOALS

Saturday

WORKOUT	MEALS	GOALS

Sunday

WORKOUT	MEALS	GOALS

Workout PLANNER

Week .... Month ....

	WORKOUT	MEALS	GOALS
Monday			

	WORKOUT	MEALS	GOALS
Tuesday			

	WORKOUT	MEALS	GOALS
Wednesday			

	WORKOUT		GOALS
Thursday			

	WORKOUT	MEALS	GOALS
Friday			

	WORKOUT	MEALS	GOALS
Saturday			

	WORKOUT	MEALS	GOALS
Sunday			

Workout PLANNER

Week .... *Month* ....

	WORKOUT	MEALS	GOALS
Monday			
Tuesday			
Wednesday			
Thursday			
Friday			
Saturday			
Sunday			

Workout PLANNER

Week .... *Month* ....

	WORKOUT	MEALS	GOALS
Monday			

	WORKOUT	MEALS	GOALS
Tuesday			

	WORKOUT	MEALS	GOALS
Wednesday			

	WORKOUT		GOALS
Thursday			

	WORKOUT	MEALS	GOALS
Friday			

	WORKOUT	MEALS	GOALS
Saturday			

	WORKOUT	MEALS	GOALS
Sunday			

Workout PLANNER

Week .... *Month* ....

	WORKOUT	MEALS	GOALS
Monday			

	WORKOUT	MEALS	GOALS
Tuesday			

	WORKOUT	MEALS	GOALS
Wednesday			

	WORKOUT	MEALS	GOALS
Thursday			

	WORKOUT	MEALS	GOALS
Friday			

	WORKOUT	MEALS	GOALS
Saturday			

	WORKOUT	MEALS	GOALS
Sunday			

Workout PLANNER

Week .... Month ....

	WORKOUT	MEALS	GOALS
Monday			

	WORKOUT	MEALS	GOALS
Tuesday			

	WORKOUT	MEALS	GOALS
Wednesday			

	WORKOUT		GOALS
Thursday			

	WORKOUT	MEALS	GOALS
Friday			

	WORKOUT	MEALS	GOALS
Saturday			

	WORKOUT	MEALS	GOALS
Sunday			

Week .... *Month* ....

	WORKOUT	MEALS	GOALS
Monday			

	WORKOUT	MEALS	GOALS
Tuesday			

	WORKOUT	MEALS	GOALS
Wednesday			

	WORKOUT		GOALS
Thursday			

	WORKOUT	MEALS	GOALS
Friday			

	WORKOUT	MEALS	GOALS
Saturday			

	WORKOUT	MEALS	GOALS
Sunday			

Workout PLANNER

Week .... Month ....

Monday	WORKOUT	MEALS	GOALS

Tuesday	WORKOUT	MEALS	GOALS

Wednesday	WORKOUT	MEALS	GOALS

Thursday	WORKOUT		GOALS

Friday	WORKOUT	MEALS	GOALS

Saturday	WORKOUT	MEALS	GOALS

Sunday	WORKOUT	MEALS	GOALS

Workout PLANNER

Week _____________   *Month* _____________

Monday	WORKOUT	MEALS	GOALS

Tuesday	WORKOUT	MEALS	GOALS

Wednesday	WORKOUT	MEALS	GOALS

Thursday	WORKOUT		GOALS

Friday	WORKOUT	MEALS	GOALS

Saturday	WORKOUT	MEALS	GOALS

Sunday	WORKOUT	MEALS	GOALS

Workout PLANNER

Week .... Month ....

	WORKOUT	MEALS	GOALS
Monday			

	WORKOUT	MEALS	GOALS
Tuesday			

	WORKOUT	MEALS	GOALS
Wednesday			

	WORKOUT		GOALS
Thursday			

	WORKOUT	MEALS	GOALS
Friday			

	WORKOUT	MEALS	GOALS
Saturday			

	WORKOUT	MEALS	GOALS
Sunday			

www.ingramcontent.com/pod-product-compliance
Lightning Source LLC
Chambersburg PA
CBHW050815260726
48660CB00004B/1434